THE MAGIC OF MOTHERHOOD

*The Story Of How A Mother Keep Her Kids Safe
By Embracing A Higher Power*

QUANG DO

Table of Contents

About the Author

Motherhood is an exciting journey where we watch our kids grow and blossom into astounding human beings. We guide them as best as we can and are awed by every milestone they achieve.

But motherhood is not always sunshine and rainbows. Sometimes, there are rainclouds and rough patches. There is worry, doubt and uncertainty.

When Quang Do gave birth to her second child, something went wrong. She suffered from severe depression and terrible anxiety. She became over-protective and fearful, and some days, she did not have the energy to get out of bed or take a shower. Every day, she hears the news about the happenings that occur all over the globe: wars, accidents, terrorisms, disasters, diseases, covid-19, deaths... She wondered why these terrible things still happened in this modern world?

There is so much that is wrong on this planet and the future promises to be filled with even more uncertainty. This is the environment that the kids of today have to grow up in and the future has to look forward to. Quang wants so much that this for her kids. She wants all their days to be filled with happiness and for them to never know an ounce of worry. And so, she worried and she fretted over things she has no chance of changing.

She tried to cope, but she spent a lot of time in a state of bewilderment. How does this work? How can my child survive all the tribulations that the world has to offer? How can I withstand the almost impossible demands of being a mother? How can I make sure that everything is and continues to be just perfect?

She feels a connection with these other women and as such, she wants to help shed light on the difficulties they go through. This book is like a transparent revelation that shares the mental, physical and emotional demands that mothers go through, especially if this woman suffers from postpartum depression. It reveals the things that mothers feel and think. It tells of the difficult periods that every mother goes through. It discloses the ways that the author has overcome the difficult postpartum depression period to unlock the power of the universe and gain happiness in the present.

This is her story.

This is my story…

Introduction

When I was expecting my first child, I had this idea about what motherhood was going to be like. I think it is par the course of becoming a mother – daydreaming, wondering and maternal preoccupancy. I created a perfect picture of motherhood with my mental musings.

I imagined taking care of my baby. My baby would coo and nurse delightful. It was a clean and ordered affair. I envisioned that while he slept, clean, dry and happy, I would make our house a beautiful home. I would clean and do laundry without interruption. I would bake and cook delicious meals, filling the house with tasty scents. I would catch up on my reading and indulge in self-care effortlessly. I would be full of energy and delight in maternal bliss. Life was going to be like a dream.

Nothing prepared me for the reality. After my first child was born, I never had this vision of a life of peace and beautiful tranquility again. Instead, I was running around in dirty clothes stained with spit, milk and baby throw up. My baby screamed for nourishment, to be changed, for attention... The list seemed endless. I spent most of my time cleaning up and caring for my baby and so, I always ran out of time before I could cook a great meal or decorate the house. I was constantly sleep-deprived and was running on fumes.

When my second baby was born, it all just became a blur. I thought having one child to care for was tough but it was nothing compared to having the pair under my wing. I did the washing, cleaned the house and fed baby number two while baby number one was still asleep. That occurred during the forgiving times, which were few and far between. Other times, they would both be awake and needing different things at the same time. I had to change the one baby while I fed the other. I would make beds while still trying to convince them to take a nap. I never worked so hard before in my life.

It is hard to reach out for help even when it is available. To let it be known that I do not have it all together because even before giving birth, most moms feel the pressure that mommy knows everything. Mommy is the magic hand that caters to all of the babies' needs. Mommy is the one that dishes out help rather than receives it.

I had to put on a brave smile and pretend to be in full control. I had to know it all. I had to understand how to stop the baby from crying and make the hurt go away when a knee was scratched or a tummy hurt. I had to know the secret remedies for taking away all maladies. I had to keep the house in check and transform the babies' tears into a giggle at the drop of a hat. That is what I thought.

After nine hours of back-breaking labor, my husband would come home and flop into a chair and complain about how tired he was. Then my second job would start. I had to care for my husband, too. He had needs. He wanted love, care and attention, and he deserved it, too.

I cared and catered for the needs of my family from the time I opened my eyes in the morning to the time I closed my eyes at night. I usually only made it until just after supper. Then I would collapse, like a dead woman. I would be out for the count.

I am a lucky woman. My husband understood how tough it was on me and he temporarily took over caring for the kids while I had a hot bath and a few minutes of self-care. I needed to pamper myself during those precious minutes if I wanted to survive the late shift.

Soon my husband would be snoring and I would be up again, feeding and baby watching. A mom's job never stops. Nor does a wife's work.

The hardest part for me was not the labor. It was a labor of love, after all. It was the image of being a perfect mother and a perfect wife. It seemed to me that I always had to be perfect. And it felt like I was failing miserably at achieving that standard of perfection.

I needed to look after my health, lose weight after my pregnancy and be a companion to my husband. I need to do it all without showing any weakness. I had to be perfect in all ways at all times. But that was an impossible dream when I was running around like a madwoman in the mornings. And when the babies were crying for one reason or another. And when I did not know how to survive even the next hour with all my babies fussing and screaming and the phone was ringing and someone is at the front door and…

I found solace in my mommy-friends. In sharing. In being able to talk – *really* talk - about anything; about incontinence and painful breasts and demanding husbands and babies that scream until they get their way. We talked about not having much time to ourselves, not even to go to the bathroom. We talked about not recognizing the new bodies we had after giving birth and coming to grips with the fact that those bodies would never be like they were before. We talked about feeling like we lost some of our identities after we became mothers. We talked about how hard it was to regain remnants of the people we were outside of being a mother.

We all went through some of the same and different tribulations. Sharing made us laugh at each other and at ourselves. It made us feel connected and allowed us to know that we were not in this mothering conundrum all alone. It allowed us to reminisce of times from the past and share our dreams and goals for the future. It allowed us to stay grounded at the moment and be present. That connection healed me and strengthened me.

Bringing kid one into the world was a roller coaster ride but having kid two was the sent me into a roller spin. My mind was my biggest enemy. Dealing with depression and anxiety, I agonized over everything. What if the kids were in an accident? What if war came to where we lived? What would I do if finances become a burden? How would I be able to protect them in case of a natural disaster? Why does Coronavirus suddenly appear in this world and quickly become the most terrible thing? How to protect my kids from the Coronavirus pandemic?

My mind was fueled into an unhealthy whirlwind and every time I heard more bad news of what was happening in the world with war, terrorism, natural disasters, floods, fires and earthquakes, the fire was fed.

I realized that people are very weak compared to the power of nature. My realization led to me finding a power that can indeed protect my kids from those bad things.

With this book, I would like to share this power with you. Let's talk, no holds barred, about the trials and tribulations, and about the profound joys that come with motherhood.

Motherhood is the greatest gift any woman can receive, and therefore, it is the most significant burden you can ever carry. I hope that your load will feel lighter when you see yourself in me, and when you realize that my stories are your stories.

I hope that you spend a little time to read to the end of this short book. This book is not only about the feelings that come with being a mom but also a sharing of how to unlock a power which can give all moms and kids the safety and happiness that rightly deserve. It is great to become a mother and you deserve to witness your children healthy and happy for the whole of this life.

Chapter One: Happiness & Bliss

Day One

After my first child was born, I was in a state of absolute bliss. I read somewhere that a woman's body is flooded with hormones like oxytocin, the love hormone that makes us connect with others, after giving birth. While I do believe that biology helps solidify that maternal bond between mother and child, I also believe that on an instinctual level mothers become connected with their babies from the moment that the seed is planted within us. No matter how the bond forms, meeting my baby was the most joyous time of my life up until then.

Love Him to Death

All I wanted to do was to look at my child. And hold my child. And caress my child. And breastfeed my child. And change my baby. And play with my baby. And make my baby laugh. And make my baby healthy.

And smile. I smiled a lot. At my husband and at all the people who came to see *my baby*. I could hardly believe he was truly mine and how perfect he was. No one else has ever had such a beautiful child. I heard one of the nurses say that. I swear.

Truly Intense Emotions

When I met my first child for the first time, I experienced the biggest wave of emotion. It felt overwhelming but so gratifying. I thought that was the pinnacle of what I was capable of feeling. Surely nothing could top that culmination.

I was wrong.

As time went on, I experienced emotions I never knew I was capable of feeling. There were huge jumps to massive joy then terrible falls to fear. There was also pride, joy and the deepest affection. When I tickled his tummy and he gurgled with laughter, I had a momentary understanding of the meaning of life. When I saw him play and interact with new things, I could make sense of everything. The whole universe just made sense when worry did not cloud my mind and I allowed myself to just observe and interact with my child. That is how deep the well of my emotion for this small human went.

Sharing With My Baby

It was a surreal thing yet so simplistic – reading to my baby. We see visions of it all the time in movies and commercials. A mother sitting on a chair with her baby on her lap and reading to the infant.

I did not appreciate how such a simple act could be so deeply connective until I did it with my own child. When I read to my son, it was more than just about developing his IQ and intelligence. When I held him and mouthed the simple words in the children's books, I could feel the softness of his skin and smell the shampoo I used in his hair. Sometimes the strands would tickle my chin when he moved or rested against me. I loved watching the deep concentration on his face as he studied the words on the page or watched the way my lips moved to pronounce them. By contrast, I also loved it when he began to dose off and his eyes lost their focus and became clouded with the need for sleep.

Even now, when I reminisce about those times, it touches a chord within me. How I loved telling him stories! As if it was just yesterday, I can clearly remember us sitting on the carpet in his room as we indulged in our usual routine. I would tickle him and he would wave his hands. After we had had a little fun, I would settle him down and I would tell him about the mouse and the elephant, or the orange orangutan who went to space. It did not matter what we read about. I just enjoyed the way he would giggle, clap and play along even though he had no idea what I am on about yet.

Watching My Baby Become a Real Person

When I had my baby, I viewed him as a baby. I did not realize until later that the way I perceived him did not really translate to a human with human tendencies, habits and a personality to me.

I remember the moment I was forced to see him differently clearly…

I heard him one afternoon. He was mimicking the mommy sounds I make when I put him to bed and had not realized that I had snuck up on him. I felt a burst of emotion seeing him imitate me. He was learning and he was evolving and it was possible through my example.

There was another moment when I found him stroking the neighbor's cat and tickling its stomach. He was showing love to the feline the way his mommy does with him. I could not hold back the tears. It was one of the most beautiful moments of my life.

Those moments altered my perception and I saw that my son was a person with thoughts and emotions that were independent of mine. He was someone with a will of his own and more than just a baby.

A Mother's Duty and Her Pride

There were times I could not help but marvel at this little human that my body sheltered and nourished for nine months. The first time he lifted his head on his own. When he learned to crawl then stand on his own two feet. How he babbled and the way his eyes lit up when he had full conversations with me in his own baby language. The first time he ate solid food… There are so many milestones, big and small, that he accomplished and every time, it was like I was hit right in the chest. The feelings of pride I felt were so strong and I knew I would never trade my mother's duty for anything despite the challenges that came with being a mother.

As he got older and smarter, I am so fulfilled and so in love with my child and his potential. I wanted to teach him everything he needs to know to make his life as accomplished as possible. I want my little man to be the greatest little man in the world. The love of a mother for her child, for her son, can surely not be equaled anywhere in creation.

Chapter Two: Panic and Fear

Depression

The depression first came for me during the night. I woke up crying softly. I think I cried for myself. I felt dead inside yet the pain in my chest told me I was quite alive. I remember wondering what the point of it all was. Everything that I do every day was surely meaningless when I am going to die one day.

Then I realized that I would not be the only one to die one day.

The realization left me feeling numb, then crippled with panicked sensations.

One day, my baby would die, too.

I started crying again. It was hard to breathe and my mind was a mess of incomplete thoughts.

My husband slept next to me, snoring softly and oblivious to the trauma I was going through.

One day my husband would die as well.

We are all going to die.

I felt the darkness enveloping me and all I wanted to do was get away.

I got up and tried to wipe the tears away. I dragged my heavy feet to the baby's room. I was so tired I could barely walk.

I watched my baby sleep and the desperate thoughts escalated. I could not handle it. Being a mom. Having the burden of these heavy thoughts. I desperately wanted to give him back. Return to sender. I made a mistake bringing him into the world. I was not fit to keep him safe and happy. Surely there was a way to send him back where he came from, right? He was so small and tender and innocent. So very vulnerable. This world was no place for him.

I had no idea how long I stood there with my heavy contemplations when I finally dragged myself back to bed, I felt angry with my husband. I was livid, in fact. Who told him he could sleep all this time, while I fought this huge war inside? Why was he not awake and vigilant and worried and busy like I was? Why was I the only one that understood the colossal mistake we made?

Anxiety

Over time I became used to feeling broken and helpless. Well, as much as a person can get used to this. The only thing that energized me as time went on was anxiety. This was a new experience. I never suffered from anxiety and now it became my unpleasant and unpredictable daily companion.

At times, it was debilitating. The constant heaviness of my thoughts made me feel like it was useless trying to get anything done. This manifested in a physical way. My limbs felt heavy, making it almost impossible to move. It was a task just getting out of bed in the morning and getting through the day grew increasingly difficult. The things I did with ease before were no longer easy to do and I was left feeling depleted of all my energy almost as soon as the day started. I was constantly detached yet restless.

Then there were the times that the anxiety fueled me into a frenzy of activity. I felt like a ticking time bomb. My thoughts were running a million miles per hour with all the things I needed to get done and it reflected in my actions. I was pulled in several directions at the same time and felt like no matter how much I accomplished there was still a growing to-do list with thousands of items that were left unticked.

My anxiety kept me up at night. I tossed and turned. My brain felt like a light bulb that could not be switched off. By the time morning rolled around, I was exhausted and all I wanted to do all day was sleep.

Panic Attack

I remember my first panic attack. I sat on the floor next to the baby's cot. His bed was too low, I suddenly thought. If there was a tsunami or even a storm, he might drown in his little bed. I sprang up and ran out of the house to get supplies and back again. I had to get his bed higher up. When my husband arrived, he said nothing. He just shook his head and removed the bricks from under the feet of the bed.

Even though he said nothing, I was burdened with the weight of his judgement.

"What's wrong with you?" his eyes said and I exploded.

I felt an overwhelming surge of panic. I felt as if I was going crazy and I wondered indeed what *was* wrong with me. I knew something was wrong but I could not for the life of me pinpoint what it was.

My chest hurt and my heart was beating too fast and too hard. I felt as if I was choking and I could not pull breath into my lungs. I trembled uncontrollably. I truly thought I would become unhinged at that moment and in my panic, I took out my frustrations on my husband.

Snakes and Scorpions

My thoughts deteriorated further after that. The fear of snakes reared its head. What if a snake slithered into the room and coiled up in my baby's bed? What if it winded around his neck or sank its fangs into him. The mental image of these things happening drove me insane with fear and for a while, I carried a stick in the house wherever I went.

I also have images of a scorpion scampering into his bed. I needed some jasmine plants to put on the windowsill. I read somewhere they repelled scorpions, but did they work on spiders too?

What If My Baby Slipped Out of the Lot and Onto the Highway?

When I had to leave my child to go to town or to a doctor's appointment, I went through seven kinds of hell. There was an incident that stands out in my mind. On my way to the funeral of one of my mom's friends, I had such a panic attack. It was so severe that we had to turn back and go home.

I had visions of my child crawling on all fours and making cute baby sounds as he tried to cross the enormous highway behind our house. I could see a big truck coming and then I imagined a plop sound, similar to a champagne cork popping. Only the presence of my husband stopped me from getting sick.

I Must Isolate My Child from the Ugliness in the World

I started to avoid the news and covered the television with a sheet. My thoughts escalated passed snakes and scorpions and deadly highways. There was danger everywhere and in everything. From the smallest utensil to the air we breathe. There was so much violence everywhere. Terrorists attacked the drop of a hat and killed hundreds. People got stabbed overshoes and lesser belongings. Friends fought and even family broke up with bleed shedding in the process. The mayhem was everywhere and all I wanted to do was sit inside to guard my baby, especially when it got dark.

Famine and Violence and Poverty and…

There was always news of children and families that were deprived of clean water and food no matter how much I tried to avoid it. What would happen if the famine came to our doorstep? My husband could lose his job at any time. Job security was a thing of the past. Surely it could happen to us, too? And what then? How would we care for a baby and buy him food and clothes and milk and toys and all the other things a child needed?

We must save more. We must be more frugal. We must… The list of musts grew every day.

Oh No, He Can Die in His Sleep

Above all, I feared that my lovely child might just die during the night. I often heard about babies dying as they sleep. Crib death is what they call it. While my world was black with depression and fear, I must have gotten up at least ten times every night to check if he was still breathing.

A few times, my heart raced when I did not see his chest move up and down or when I did not hear the soft puff of air leave his nose. He is dead, I would think. My eyes would already be moist before I heard the soft inhales and exhales. He was alive! My joy was intense. For a moment… Then the bleakness would return.

Chapter Three: Difficulties and Desperations

Giving Birth is Painful

I thought things could not get worse. Then my second child was born…

The labor was terrible. I am not sure if it was worse than my first labor. Even my mommy-friends concurred that the pain of labor became a distant memory after all was said and done. But this time around, the pain stuck with me. I suspect it was because I was already in a bad mental state.

I remembered being at the hospital as the contractions grew more and more painful. The pain radiated around my thighs, midsection and back. I felt cold and hot at the same time. Deep breathing did not seem to help.

I had to throw away my lovely pajamas and opted for the hospital's gown instead. There was lots of sweat and the other bodily fluids that came with delivering a child.

The aftermath was not much better than the delivery. Everything continued to hurt. My breasts were swollen and tender, and my nipples squirted milk. It seemed like I was permanently covered in milk. I was overwhelmed and all I wanted to do was pause time and remove myself for just a little while so I could get my bearings.

But that was impossible and every task I performed reminded me of that. Even going to the bathroom… The nurse often had to come to the bathroom with me with a bottle of water to get things going and I had to use the softest pads in the world just to pamper my broken parts after taking a pee.

Tantrums and Hysterics

The first few days at home after my second delivery was a test of my mantle. My body felt sluggish and nothing seemed to work as well after he was born. Sometimes, my boy would throw a tantrum. He would kick with his hands and feet. His face would red with anger and he screamed and cried all the time. I think he went on crying unabatedly for three days. He simply could not stop crying, and I had to bite my hand not to really lose my temper for this little angry person.

It only made things worse that my worries were centered around two children now instead of one.

Utter Exhaustion

Every time, just as I fell asleep, kid 2 would start to bawl again. And I could hear him crying harder and harder as he went along without attention. I would feed him and change him, and just as I fall asleep, he would go off again. He was terrorizing me, I swear.

I tried the typically coping mechanisms that all the professionals recommended. I breathed in and out deeply. I tried counting softly. When those techniques did not work, I decided to pretend not to mind but it was a hard battle. I am not naturally patient so I had to really work at it.

No Time for My Chores

Maintaining a house with one kid underfoot was difficult but doing it with two was almost impossible. It was tough to cook or do the washing, or anything else that did not relate to caring for the baby. Most of the time I just had to leave it all as it was to tend to the baby's never-ending needs. He needed a bath. He needed a bottle. He needed a dummy. He needed a nap. It never stopped. I became very, very tired over time.

Feeding, Spitting and Refusal to Eat

When it comes to nutrition, I was fortunate. He was always hungry and soon went onto solids. The unfortunate way was that he became very picky the moment he started eating solids. He would simply spit out anything he disliked. I had to duck and struggled to remain patient and calm enough to persuade him not to behave like a little barbarian.

Patience and Discipline

It was hard to understand how far I should go. Should I always give him his way? Wouldn't he end up spoiled if I did? It often became a battle of the minds: his unfettered demands versus my continuing struggle to draw the line. It made me exhausted, and I had some of the worst fights with my husband, ever, about this.

Whenever he was around, he wanted to please the child and then my attempt at discipline went out of the window. We had some furious rows about this issue.

Chapter Four: Solace and Solutions

When confronted with what seems to be an insurmountable problem, we have one of two choices: innovate or run. That's it. And these were the options I had when it all came crashing down.

I simply could not keep it up.

Between the emotional upheavals and the drama between the chores and my responsibilities to my husband and children, I knew I had to change if I wanted to survive as a wife and mother.

For a while, as I contemplated the difficulties and dramas of motherhood, my inner voice tried to break through but somehow I could never hear it clearly.

All of this changed when my eldest son cut his foot open to the bone.

The boys were playing outside when they found a glass bottle in a ditch and decided to break the glass. When their friends arrived, my youngest smashed the bottle and there was glass everywhere. He cleverly warned his friends not to cut themselves and subsequently stepped on a sharp piece and cut his foot severely. He bled profusely.

Just like any normal child that age, he cried and screamed. Hearing his painful pleas almost sent my head in to a tizzy. At the sight of all that blood, I felt like all my fears were becoming reality.

I wanted to panic but this was the moment I finally heard my own inner voice. It cut through all the other thoughts and it instructed me. Hearing it helped me to remain calm. I phoned my husband and he promised to be there as soon as he could. While I waited for him, I put my son in a tub and tried to stop the bleeding. My husband arrived not long after. We took our son to the local hospital and he was stitched and bandaged. We were lucky there were no complications.

That moment changed everything.

While I would never wish ill on my own child, I needed that moment to help me see clearly. My own voice came to life. I could now hear my inner-self admonishing me about all my unfounded fears and worries. The voice forced me to look into myself rather than worry about the externalities I could not control. I realized that it was all about faith. First off, I had to trust in nature. In human nature. I was a woman and I was equipped to be a mother. It was something that we humans can naturally do. When I understood that, the battle was half won.

There is more to it, though. It is also about the realization of limits. By understanding that I was as good as any mom in the world, it also became clear to me that I was, therefore, as limited as any human being in the world, too.

We need help from outside ourselves if we want to become our best selves. I had my husband and family for support and for too long, I pushed them away. I handled the accident calmly. When I realized that my son was severely hurt, I was calm enough to be rational. I put him in a washbasin. I phoned my husband. I hugged the bleeding child. I assured him mommy was going to make things better. And I called the hospital. I understood that I had to help myself to get help from my husband and the medical staff at the hospital.

When I contemplate that afternoon, I realize that it ended my focus on myself. Instead of being obsessed with my problems, my work, my chores, my fears and my anxieties, I suddenly changed my focus and concentrated on only my sons.

My insight led me to a more profound sense of faith and a thirst for more understanding. Over time I came to understand that I – as all moms do - have the power inside. All I had to do was to learn how to unlock that power for the sake of my own happiness and the safety and security of my family.

This is what MEDICINE BUDDHA is all about. When you feel small and helpless, when you feel the desire to pray, remind yourself of the power of Medicine Buddha. It is only through the strength of His mantras that I developed the ability to ultimately unlock my own strength and to protect my children and my husband from my fears and anxiety. If you project your doubts on the people you love, you bring misfortune to their lives and to your own.

Chapter Five: Who Gives Us The Power?

To survive my perilous journey as a young mother, I found solace in my friends, family and in some of the wisdom of the ages. I prayed. I joined many social media groups. And finally, I decided to learn about universe's power.

We have heard the magnetic field. We have heard the invisible waves of all kinds. They are invisible but they have the power. And in this universe, how many such magic and invisible powers still exist?

Why is the Earth spinning? Why is the moon orbiting the earth? Why is there a tide? Why is there day and night?

These things happen because there is an invisible force propelling them into action. Certainly, there are still intangible things that exist in this universe. And certainly, universe contains many great and magic powers, including Gods and Buddhas. But where are Lords in this world and how can they hear our prayer? How to get response from them? I read many books. I read many Buddha sutras to find out the answer for those questions.

The Medicine Buddha always watches over sentient beings in their lives. He give them peace, happiness and freedom from diseases and other sufferings.

It doesn't matter if you are Christian, Buddhist or nonreligious, Medicine Buddha is your PROTECTOR who always protect you and your family. He is not only a Buddha but also a Doctor who can cure all our problems, bad karmas, sufferings and diseases.

In His Sutra book ("Sutra of the Medicine Buddha"), in His seventh vow, He stated that: *"...those who are tormented by diseases, who have nobody to whom they can seek for help, without a refuge, without a doctor, without medicine, without relatives, without a home; these poor and miserable beings shall all of them be free from diseases and troubles, and shall enjoy perfect health of body and mind, once my name reaches their ears. They shall have families, friends and properties a-plenty,..."*

He also stated in His twelve vow: *"all beings who are poor and naked, tormented day and night by mosquitoes and wasps, by cold and heat, when they hear my name and carefully remember and cherish it, shall receive the wonderful garments of all kinds, as well as valuable ornaments, chaplets of fragrant flower; and various kinds of instrumental music shall resound. Whatever they dream of, they shall have in abundance."*

He said, *"I proved beyond any doubt that all your requests, all your dreams will come true."*

Where of this universe is He? How to make your prayer to reach Him?

Just calling His name in this mantra: "Namo Medicine Buddha". Please repeat "Namo Medicine Buddha" more than 1080 times per day, and then, pray for the safety and health of your family. It's not only a praying. It's a mantra! Remember to close your eyes and focus your mind on each word of this mantra. Believe absolutely in His power, this power will work for your praying.

This is where I go when I face adversity, when my fears paralyze me and when my anxiety makes it hard to function. I say, "Namo Medicine Buddha."

This is his power. This is my power. This is your power. This is our power. This is the way to unlock your strengths and to become the best version of yourself.

This power is for all people. This mantra is for all people.

"Namo Medicine Buddha."

Conclusion: Keep the Magic

The hardest part of being a mother is to draw a line in the sand – to understand where you end and where your child begins. No matter how close you feel to them, rearing children means breaking the link, severing the connection at some point and allowing them to become individuals apart from yourself.

During this journey, as a mother, you live in fear of loss and failure. A mother's life is, in that sense, a life filled with loss.

It would be great if all moms realize that there was no one path that led to being a great mother. I realized that I am not have to be perfect nor did the act of mothering have to be perfect. And I learned to accept the things I had no control over and do my best at the things I did have control over. I realized that I did not have to stack my abilities and performance up to another mother to find validation in those abilities and performance.

It is only after you make peace with loss and failure and give yourself over to a higher power that you will unlock your deepest reserves. Only then can you become a super-mom and live to love your children. Now I spend a little time per day to repeat Medicine Buddha's mantra. Let our minds peaceful and let Him protect all of us.

"Namo Medicine Buddha."

www.ingramcontent.com/pod-product-compliance
Lightning Source LLC
Chambersburg PA
CBHW051141250726
48655CB00007B/3173